Homemade Waterproof Sunscreen:

20 Kid-Friendly Sunscreen Recipes with SPF 15 And Higher

I0413988

Table of content

Book introduction

Homemade sunscreens are a great way to benefit your family and children and keep them away from those sunscreens that are available in the supermarkets. Not only these sunscreens are loaded with chemicals they are also extremely overpriced. Little of them might be real the rest is all artificial.

It is better to make sunscreens at home in the natural and easy way. SPF is another important factor to consider when making sunscreens at home. SPF stands for sun protection factor which means the higher an ingredient has SPF the more affective it is in preventing your skin from burning.

Following the note on SPF it is better to use those ingredients which have a higher SPF so that you benefit from these sunscreens in the maximum possible way. Some of the ingredients which have a great SPF include, carrot seed oil, red raspberry oil, raw unrefined coconut oil and ofcourse zinc oxide which has the highest SPF factor.

With the help of this information you can look in for those ingredients which have higher SPF and buy those specially when you go to buy. Some essential oils have also been added which not only give fragrance to your sunscreens but are also good for your skin.

The other ingredients such as the oils, jojoba oil, coconut oil, olive oil, shea butter, beeswax all are beneficial and healthy for your skin and benefit your skin in some way or another. Learn the correct method of these sunscreens and make them at your home!

Recipe 01: Whipped shea butter sunscreen

Description: Shea butter has a SPF of approximately 5 – 6 which will aid in giving protection from the sun but just the shea butter is not enough to give complete protection from the sun which is why a few more ingredients are added.

The addition of zinc oxide in this recipe will give a SPF of around 40+ and without the zinc oxide the SPF will be somewhere between 20 to 30 so it is recommended to add the zinc oxide as the more the SPF the better the protection from the sun.

Ingredients:

- Shea butter- ½ cup
- Melted coconut oil- 1/3 cup
- Carrot seed essential oil- 15 to 16 drops, has a SPF of 40.
- Myrrh essential oil- 10 to 11 drops
- Zinc oxide- 2 drops, has a SPF of 20.

Recipe:

- Measure all the ingredients carefully or else a slight mistake will not make the sunscreen to be fluffy.
- Whip the raw shea butter until it is fluffy and creamy.
- Melt the coconut oil.
- Now add the coconut oil to the shea butter while whipping it.
- Now add the carrot seed essential oil.
- Add in the myrrh essential oil and mix.
- Now add the zinc oxide without inhaling and whip.
- Whip until fluffy and pour in to bottle.
- Now the sunscreen is ready to be applied.

Recipe 02: Homemade tea tree essential oil sunscreen

Description: This homemade sunscreen smells really pleasant because of the tea tree essential oil added to it. This homemade tea tree essential oil has a SPF of about 20 and is the perfect sunscreen you can use to apply on your kids.

This recipe makes water proof sunscreen bars that can be refrigerated once you are done using them and once they are used. You can refrigerate them and then take them out when you wish to use them.

Ingredients:

- Beeswax- 1.5 oz
- Shea butter- 1.5 oz
- Coconut oil- 1.5 oz
- Zinc oxide- 1 oz
- Tea tree oil- about 10 drops

Recipe:

- Measure all the ingredients properly to be precise and accurate as a slight mistake can change the consistency of your sunscreen.
- Take a mason jar and add in the beeswax, shea butter and the coconut oil.
- Put this mason jar in boiling water and let these 3 ingredients mix properly together.
- Remove from heat and now add in the zinc oxide.
- Now add the tea tree oil.
- Pour the mixture in to molds or in ice cube trays and refrigerate them.

- Remove from molds and use them and then refrigerate them again until you wish to use them again.

Recipe 03: DIY waterproof sunscreen

Description: This waterproof sunscreen is a natural sunscreen with some good ingredients to help you against the sun heat. It is easy to make and has the ingredients with a good Sun protection factor.

The sweet almond oil added is great for skin elasticity. Here is how you should make it.

Ingredients:

- Coconut oil- ½ cup, has a SPF of 10.
- Sweet almond oil- ¼ cup
- Beeswax- ¼ cup
- Shea butter- 2 tablespoon
- Vitamin E- 1 teaspoon
- Zinc oxide powder- 2 tablespoon, has a natural SPF of 20.
- Lavender essential oil- 3 drops

Recipe:

- In a double boiler, add the coconut oil, sweet almond oil, beeswax, shea butter and the lavender essential oil and let everything mix and incorporate.
- Remove from heat and pour in to a glass jar.
- Now add in the zinc oxide powder without inhaling.
- Put the lid on the jar and shake to mix in everything well.
- Pour in to desired containers or molds and let them cool before using.
- Use it when you are out in the sun for a long period of time.

Recipe 04: Beeswax sunscreen lotion

Description: In this sunscreen lotion recipe there are many good ingredients that can help you achieve protection from the sun. make this sunscreen lotion at home for your kids and apply on their skins for prolonged safety from the sun heat.

Ingredients:

- Wheat germ oil- 1 ounce, has a SPF of 20.
- Beeswax- 1 ounce, has a SPF of 15.
- Shea butter- 1 ounce
- Vitamin E oil- 1 teaspoon
- Zinc oxide powder- 0.36 ounces, has a SPF of 20.
- Eucalyptus essential oil- 30 drops

Recipe:

- In a double boiler, add the wheat germ oil, beeswax, shea butter and the vitamin E oil.
- Let them melt and incorporate together.
- Now add the eucalyptus essential oil and mix.
- Pour in to a mason jar.
- Now carefully add the zinc oxide powder and mix.
- Close the lid and shake to mix all the ingredients together.
- Pour it in to molds or a plastic container and let it cool before using.

Recipe 05: Homemade cocoa butter sunscreen

Description: In this recipe of homemade cocoa butter sunscreen there is cocoa butter added which gives a really good smell to the sunscreen. Cocoa butter is great for our skin and keeps it really smooth and is best for kids as they have sensitive skin.

Ingredients:

- Beeswax- 2 ounces, has a SPF of 15.
- Cocoa butter- 2 ounces
- Coconut oil- 2 ounces
- Carrot seed oil- 2 ounces, has a SPF of 40.
- Zinc oxide powder- 2 ounces, has a SPF of 20.
- Kitchen scale
- Double boiler
- Squeeze tubes

Recipe:

- Take a double boiler and melt in the beeswax, cocoa butter and the coconut oil together.
- Remove it from heat and now add in the zinc oxide powder and keep stirring it.
- Cool the mixture and now add the carrot seed oil and mix.
- Pour the liquid mixture in to squeeze tubes and close the lid.
- Apply the sunscreen on your skin and your kids when required.

Recipe 06: DIY natural SPF 40 sunblock using coconut oil, carrot seed oil and essential oil

Description: The following recipe is not only of a sunblock but it is also a chemical free and healthy solution to abstain from sunlight and getting yourselves and your children burned. This sunblock has vital nutrients and is a kind of beauty treatment for you as well.

The carrot seed oil in this recipe has a SPF of 40 which means this sunblock is an excellent source of getting yourself protected from sunlight.

Ingredients:

- Organic coconut oil- two tablespoons
- Avocado oil Organic - 1 tablespoon
- Shea butter Organic - 1 tablespoon
- Organic sesame oil- ½ teaspoon
- Carrot seed oil Organic - 30 droplets
- Aloe vera gel Organic - ½ teaspoon

Recipe:

- In a double boiler, melt the organic coconut oil and the shea butter.
- Add in the avocado oil, sesame oil and the aloe vera gel and let all the oils melt and combine together.
- Now add in the organic carrot seed oil and mix.
- Pour in to a bottle or a plastic container and let it cool.

Recipe 07: Raspberry seed oil sunscreen recipe

Description: The red raspberry seed oil has a SPF of about 28 to 50 which is why the sunscreens having raspberry seed oil are the most effective ones. The more the SPF, the more better the sunscreen is. Along with the raspberry seed oil, carrot seed oil is also added in this recipe which makes it more effective.

Ingredients:

- Coconut oil- ¼ cup
- Shea butter- ¼ cup
- Sesame oil- 1/8 cup
- Beeswax granules- 2 tablespoons
- Red raspberry seed oil- 1 teaspoon
- Carrot seed oil- 1 teaspoon

Recipe:

- With the help of the double boiler, melt the coconut oil, shea butter, sesame oil and the beeswax granules.
- After all the oils have melted then remove from heat.
- Let them cool to room temperature.
- Keep the mixture in the refrigerator for about 10 minutes.
- Remove from fridge and start whipping it with a hand mixer.
- Now add in the red raspberry seed oil and then the carrot seed oil.
- Whip until the mixture is light and fluffy,
- Store in to plastic or glass containers or in squeezable bottles and use it when required.

Recipe 08: Homemade facial sunscreen recipe

Description: In this homemade facial sunscreen recipe, jojoba oil is used which has a SPF of around 8, zinc oxide powder which has a SPF of 40 and red raspberry seed oil which has a SPF of around 28 to 50 which makes this sunscreen a very effective one.

Use this recipe to make a homemade facial sunscreen for your kids and apply to their skins whenever you go out in the sun.

Ingredients:

- Shea butter- ¼ cup
- Jojoba oil- 2 tablespoon
- Beeswax- 2 tablespoon
- Vitamin E oil- 1 teaspoon
- Red raspberry seed oil- 10 drops
- Zinc oxide powder- 1 tablespoon

Recipe:

- With the help of a double boiler, melt the shea butter, jojoba oil and the beeswax.
- The beeswax will take a long time to melt rather than the other 2.
- Let the oils melt and then remove them from heat.
- Now add in the vitamin E oil and mix.
- Next, add the red raspberry seed oil and the zinc oxide powder.
- Make sure you do not inhale the zinc oxide powder and keep your mouth covered.
- Mix properly and pour the mixture in to plastic containers or squeezable bottles.

- Let the sunscreen come on room temperature before using it.
- Use this sunscreen as you would use any sunscreen with a SPF of 30 to 40.

Recipe 09: The best waterproof homemade sunscreen

Description: Zinc oxide has a SPF of about 40 and this makes this sunscreen really effective in preventing your child's skin from burning. The other ingredients include coconut oil and beeswax both of which have a SPF of 8 and 15 respectively.

Apart from this carrot seed oil is also added in this homemade sunscreen which has a SPF of 40 which makes this sunscreen to be one of the most effective ones. You can easily make this sunscreen and apply it on your children's skins to prevent them from getting the sunlight.

Although the lavender essential oil and the myrrh essential oils used in this recipe are optional, it is advisable to use them as the lavender oil has an amazing fragrance and these essential oils are not only amazing in their fragrances but they are also good for your skins.

Ingredients:

- Coconut oil- 1 cup
- Beeswax- 4 tablespoon
- Herbal tea- 1 cup
- Non-nano zinc oxide powder- 2 oz
- Carrot seed oil- 20 drops
- Lavender essential oil- 20 drops
- Myrrh essential oil- 10 drops
- Squeeze tubes- 4 to 5.

Recipe:

- With the help of your double boiler, melt the coconut oil and the beeswax together.
- Now add in your herbal tea in the double boiler to let it mix properly.
- Cool this mixture.
- Pour the cooled mixture in to a blender and blend.
- Keep blending until the mixture is smooth.
- Now add the zinc oxide powder and be careful not to inhale.
- Next add the carrot seed oil, lavender essential oil and the myrrh essential oil.
- Mix and pour in to squeezable tubes.
- Your sunscreen is now ready to be used.

Recipe 10: Homemade beach cream

Description: All of the ingredients added in this homemade beach cream have natural SPF's added to them. This means that you are adding zero chemicals to your body. You are not only moisturizing your body but also giving the medical benefits of each ingredient to your body.

The essential oils added in this recipe have some amazing benefits for you. The carrot seed oil not only has a SPF of 28 but it is also an antioxidant which protects the skin naturally. The carrot seed oil is also great for digestive system.

The myrrh essential oil is a healing oil which is great for our skin and is known for its amazing benefits.

This homemade beach cream can be easily made as it is simple with just a few ingredients and can be applied and used for your kids.

Ingredients:

- Raw shea butter- 1 cup, has a SPF of 5.
- Coconut oil- 2/3 cup, has a SPF of 6.
- Carrot seed essential oil- 30 drops, has a SPF of 28.
- Myrrh essential oil- 20 drops, has a SPF of 15.
- Squeeze tubes- 2

Recipe:

- In a mixing bowl, add the raw shea butter and the coconut oil.
- Beat them on medium speed.
- Both should be beaten and whipped until they look like a buttery icing.
- They should be smooth and creamy.
- Now add in the carrot seed essential oil.
- Next add in the myrrh essential oil and mix.
- Pour in to squeeze tubes and your sunscreen is now ready to be applied.

Recipe 11: Chemical free DIY natural sunscreen

Description: The zinc oxide added in this sunscreen prevents from the UVA rays which is quite rare in the other supermarket sunscreens out there. This is a natural sunscreen that can be made at home and the zinc oxide has a SPF of 40 which is amazing for your child's skin as they will be heavily protected from the sun.

Coconut oil and olive oil are also used in this sunscreen recipe and both have a SPF of 8 and 15. Coconut oil has some amazing properties such as being an antioxidant, anti-inflammatory and has anti-bacterial benefits as well.

Olive oil however has a lot of vitamin E in it and is loaded with anti- aging oxidants and with its high SPF of 15 it really promotes to good skin health.

Ingredients:

- Coconut oil- 2.5 oz
- Olive oil- 1.5 oz
- Beeswax- 5 oz
- Filtered water- 4 oz
- Zinc oxide- 2 tablespoons
- Natural preservative such as liquid radish root - ½ teaspoon
- Peppermint essential oil- 6 drops

Recipe:

- With the help of a double boiler, melt the coconut oil, olive oil and the beeswax.

- The beeswax may take the longest time to melt.

- Remove from heat and add in the filtered water.

- Mix until the mixture becomes creamy.

- Now add in the zinc oxide and stir.

- Add in the natural preservative and the peppermint essential oil.

- Pour the mixture into mason jars and your sunscreen is now ready to be applied.

Recipe 12: Coconut oil sunscreen recipe

Description: Coconut oil has a natural SPF of 5 and it contains antioxidants which protect the skin from harmful radiation of the sun. Only the coconut oil is not enough for a long day in the sun which is why we add the raspberry seed oil which has a SPF of 25. Zinc oxide is also added which has a great SPF and which protects from the sunlight.

Carrot seed oil has a SPF of 28 and is also added in this sunscreen recipe.

Ingredients:

- Virgin coconut oil- ½ cup
- Non nano zinc oxide- 2 tablespoons
- Red raspberry seed oil- 1 tablespoon
- Carrot seed essential oil- 10 drops

Recipe:

- Take a food processor and add in the virgin coconut oil and mix it.
- Now add the non nano zinc oxide and be careful not to inhale it.
- Next add the red raspberry seed oil.
- Add in the carrot seed essential oil and mix all the ingredients.
- Pour the mixture in to a small container.
- Now your sunscreen is ready to be applied.

Recipe 13: Homemade shea butter sunscreen

Description: This homemade shea butter sunscreen will leave your skin to be softer than ever before. The ingredients in this sunscreen recipe will keep your kids skin nourished and heal and soften than ever before.

The coconut oil in this sunscreen recipe has a SPF of 10 as well as the shea butter.

Carrot seed oil is amazing for our skin and has a SPF of about 38 to 40. Zinc powder is also added in this sunscreen recipe and has a SPF of 20. Together combined with the other ingredients this homemade sunscreen recipe is an amazing one which you can use to apply on your kid's skins.

Ingredients:

- Coconut oil- ¼ cup
- Shea butter- 2 tablespoons
- Carrot seed oil- 2 teaspoon
- Almond oil- ¼ cup
- Zinc powder- 3 tablespoons
- Beeswax- 1 oz
- Lavender essential oil- 10 drops

Recipe:

- In a microwave safe dish, melt the coconut oil, beeswax and the shea butter.
- Stir and add in the zinc oxide powder without inhaling.
- Stir until the mixture is smooth and melted.

- Cool the mixture for a few minutes.
- After the mixture is cooled, add in the carrot seed oil and the almond oil.
- Now mix in the lavender essential oil.
- Pour the mixture in to a mason jar.
- Now your sunscreen is ready to be used.

Recipe 14: Homemade DIY sunscreen

Description: This is a chemical free recipe of a DIY homemade sunscreen that is actually excellent for your children. People who have used this sunscreen have shared amazing experiences with this sunscreen. This sunscreen is so effective that you will continue to get its benefits even after spending 8 days or more at your camp or if you spend too many hours at the beach.

This recipe is not of a chemical sunscreen instead it is packed with those ingredients who have a high SPF which means they are more efficient in preventing yourself getting burned from the sunlight.

The coconut oil in this recipe has a SPF of 10, the avocado oil has a SPF of 15, beeswax has a SPF of 15, shea butter has a SPF of 6 and zinc oxide has a SPF of 40 so this is an amazing sunscreen recipe which you must try out.

Ingredients:

- Coconut oil- 90 grams
- Avocado oil- 65 grams
- Beeswax- 28.5 grams
- Shea butter- 27.5 grams
- Zinc oxide- 40 grams
- Vitamin E- ½ teaspoon

Recipe:

- Make sure you have a mask around your mouth before starting to make this sunscreen.

- Melt the coconut oil, avocado oil, shea butter and the beeswax in a double boiler and melt all the ingredients together.

- The beeswax will take the longest time to melt.

- Stir until the mixture turns into a smooth consistency.

- Now add in the vitamin E and mix.

- Remove from heat and add in the zinc oxide slowly and gradually while making sure you do not inhale at all.

- Whisk and whisk carefully.

- Completely cool the mixture and pour it into any container of your choice.

- Leave it to set for a while and after a few minutes your sunscreen will be completely ready.

- You can now use it and apply on your skin.

- You can now use it and apply on your skin.

Recipe 15: Naturally homemade sunscreen

Description: In this natural homemade sunscreen recipe various oils have been used that have different amounts of SPF. While some have lower SPF and some have higher SPF the main difference is made by the zinc oxide which has a SPF of about 40 and which is the most effective ingredient in preventing yourself from the sun.

Carrot seed oil added in this recipe has a SPF of about 38 to 40 while shea butter has a SPF of 6. Jojoba oil also added in this recipe has a SPF of 4. These different ingredients combined together make this sunscreen very effective. You can make this sunscreen at your home and use it on your kid's skin and help them prevent from the scorching heat of the sun.

Ingredients:

- Carrot seed oil- 1 oz
- Shea butter- 0.8 oz
- Jojoba oil- 0.1 oz
- Vitamin E oil- 0.1 oz
- Lavender essential oil- 15 drops
- Eucalyptus essential oil- 10 drops
- Peppermint essential oil- 5 drops
- Zinc oxide powder- 2 oz

Recipe:

- In a double boiler, add the carrot seed oil, shea butter and the jojoba oil and let them melt.
- Heat until the shea butter is melted.

- Remove from the double boiler and let the mixture cool completely.
- Put a mask on your face so not to inhale the zinc oxide powder and slowly slowly add the zinc oxide powder.
- Add in the vitamin E oil and stir.
- Now add in the lavender essential oil. Eucalyptus essential oil and the peppermint essential oil and stir to mix in all the ingredients.
- Pour the cooled mixture in to your desired container and let it set for a few minutes.
- Now your sunscreen is ready to be applied.
- Store it in the refrigerator after use.

Recipe 16: Non-toxic homemade sunscreen with wheatgerm

Description: Wheat germ has a SPF of 20 and the higher the SPF the more affective your sunscreen will be. Apart from wheatgerm, raw unrefined coconut oil is used in this recipe in its solid form which has a SPF of 10 to 20.

Jojoba oil and, olive oil and shea butter are also added in this recipe. Although they have good properties and can prevent the skin from the sunlight just these are not enough and it is necessary to add in such an ingredient which has a high SPF than these.

This non-toxic homemade sunscreen is great for kids and even teenagers can use it. It is simple to make with a few simple ingredients.

Ingredients:

- Raw and unrefined coconut oil- 2 cups
- Wheat germ oil- ½ cup
- Olive oil- 1/8 cup
- Hazelnut oil- 1/8 cup
- Jojoba oil- 1/8 cup
- Shea butter- ½ cup
- Eucalyptus essential oil- 20 drops

Recipe:

- Put half of the unrefined coconut oil in a bowl and beat and whip it with a stand mixer.

- Now add in the wheat germ oil, olive oil. Hazelnut oil, shea butter and the jojoba oil.

- Beat until the mixture turns smooth and creamy.

- Start putting in the eucalyptus essential oil slowly and gradually starting from a few drops.

- Now add the rest of the coconut oil and beat to form a smooth mixture.

- Pour the mixture in to a jar and let it set for a few minutes.

- Your sunscreen is now ready to be applied.

- Rub on exposed skin and rub it well.

- Apply 10 minutes before going out in the sunlight.

Recipe 17: Homemade cocoa butter sunscreen recipe

Description: Cocoa butter has a SPF of 15 and it is excellent for our skin. It gives the skin a smooth and soft texture and has an amazing fragrance as well. Apart from this, zinc oxide powder is also added which has a SPF of 40. Wheatgerm oil has a SPF of 20 which makes it really affective when added to sunscreens. This sunscreen is very easy to make and you can easily make it at your home.

Ingredients:

- Carrot seed oil- 1 ounce
- Cocoa butter- 1 ounce
- Vitamin E oil-1 teaspoon
- Zinc oxide powder- 0.36 ounces
- Lavender essential oil- 15 drops
- Peppermint essential oil- 15 drops

Recipe:

- In a double boiler, melt the carrot seed oil and the cocoa butter.
- Remove from heat and add in the vitamin E oil.
- Cover your mouth so you do not inhale and add in the zinc oxide powder slowly.
- Let the mixture cool and add in the lavender essential oil and the peppermint essential oil.
- Pour the mixture in to any desired container and let it set for a few minutes.
- Now your sunscreen is ready to be applied.
- This sunscreen is best for kids aged till 10.

Recipe 18: Pomegranate sunscreen

Description: In this sunscreen recipe, pomegranate oil is used which not only has a good fragrance but also has some good properties. Zinc oxide is added as well as it has a good SPF and helps in protection from the sun.

Coconut oil and shea butter are also added both of which have SPF of 8 and 6 respectively. This sunscreen is easy to make and has just a few ingredients.

Ingredients:

- Lavender essential oil- 10 drops
- Pomegranate oil- 1 tablespoon
- Coconut oil- ¾ cup
- Zinc oxide- 2 tablespoon
- Shea butter- 2 tablespoon

Recipe:

- In a double boiler, add the pomegranate oil, coconut oil and the shea butter and let it melt.
- Remove from heat and add in the lavender essential oil.
- Slowly add in the zinc oxide powder and be careful not to inhale in.
- Mix and pour the mixture in to a glass jar and let it set for a few minutes.

Recipe 19: Homemade natural sunscreen for babies

Description: This homemade natural sunscreen has a SPF of about 30 and it is very smooth. It can rub easily on your skin and prevent your babies skin to get burned from the sunlight.

The shea butter in this recipe has a SPF of about 6 and the coconut oil has a SPF of 10. Zinc oxide has a higher SPF as compared to both of these and more zinc oxide can be added if you desire a sunscreen that has a much more higher SPF.

Adding more zinc oxide will also increase the whiteness of this sunscreen. The ingredients are simple and are easily available.

Ingredients:

- Beeswax pallets- 3 tablespoons
- Shea butter- ½ cup
- Coconut oil- ½ cup
- Zinc oxide- 4 tablespoon
- Lavender essential oil- 10 drops (optional)

Recipe:

- With the help of a double boiler, add in the beeswax pallets, shea butter and the coconut oil and melt them.
- Keep stirring continuously until they are smooth and melted.
- Remove from heat.

- Add in the zinc oxide slowly and gradually and make sure not to inhale as it can be dangerous.
- Add in the lavender essential oil if you desire.
- Pour the mixture into desired plastic containers.
- Let it set and your sunscreen is now ready to be applied.

Recipe 20: Homemade sunscreen lotion bars

Description: In this recipe, coconut oil is used which has a SPF of 10 and the shea butter has a SPF of 6. Zinc oxide is added which has a higher SPF than both and which adds whiteness to the sunscreen.

This sunscreen is exceptionally great for your babies and you can apply on their skins without having to worry about them getting burned.

Ingredients:

- melted coconut oil- 1/3 cup
- shea butter- 1/3 cup
- grated beeswax- ½ cup
- non-nano zinc oxide- 2 tablespoons plus 1.5 teaspoons
- cocoa powder for tinting- 1 teaspoon

Recipe:

- In a double boiler, melt the coconut oil, shea butter and the beeswax.
- Remove from heat and add in the zinc oxide powder and be careful not to inhale it.
- Stir until blended and now pour into molds.
- Top with the cocoa powder.
- Let them cool and set.
- Now remove from the molds and use when required.
- To apply rub on the skin and massage.

Conclusion

At the end of this book, it is now easy to say that you might have learned a great deal about how to make sunblock creams, sunblock lotions and natural sunscreens at home by using just a few common ingredients.

With the help of this book you must have learned about a variety of things such as the kind of ingredients used in making natural sunscreens and ofcourse a great deal about SPF.

It is better to learn how to make sunscreens at your home and preparing them in the natural way rather than buying the supermarket ones that although are so readily and easily available but ultimately a great concern as they are practically loaded with chemicals.

This book mentions 20 recipes of homemade sunscreens that you can use to apply on your babies and childrens skins. You must however not take this process as too easy and you should remember a few points when you make these sunscreens at home.

First, you must be familiar with the main ingredient in almost every recipe that is zinc oxide. Zinc oxide should be added carefully when you prepare your sunscreen and you should make sure not to inhale in the scent as it can be dangerous for you.

The handling of the equipments such as the double boiler and the melting of the oils should be done with great care and it is better to keep the children away when you are doing this work.

In the end, we wish you an amazing read with this book of homemade natural sunscreens!

FREE Bonus Reminder

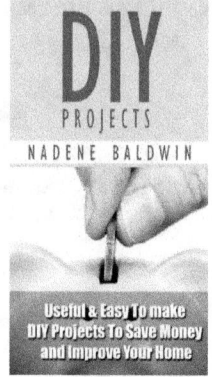

If you have not grabbed it yet, please go ahead and download your special bonus report *"DIY Projects. 13 Useful & Easy To Make DIY Projects To Save Money & Improve Your Home!"*

Simply Click the Button Below

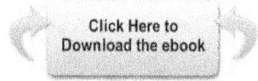

OR **Go to This Page**

http://diyhomecraft.com/free

BONUS #2: More Free & Discounted Books or Products

Do you want to receive more Free/Discounted Books or Products?

We have a mailing list where we send out our new Books or Products when they go free or with a discount on Amazon. Click on the link below to sign up for Free & Discount Book & Product Promotions.

=> **Sign Up for Free & Discount Book & Product Promotions** <=

OR Go to this URL

http://zbit.ly/1WBb1Ek

www.ingramcontent.com/pod-product-compliance
Lightning Source LLC
Chambersburg PA
CBHW061931280526
45787CB00004B/1559